YOUR KNOWLEDGE HAS VALUE

AF131197

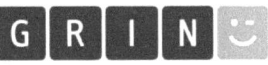

Bibliographic information published by the German National Library:

The German National Library lists this publication in the National Bibliography; detailed bibliographic data are available on the Internet at http://dnb.dnb.de .

Imprint:

Copyright © 2016 GRIN Verlag, Open Publishing GmbH
Print and binding: Books on Demand GmbH, Norderstedt Germany
ISBN: 9783668408487

This book at GRIN:

http://www.grin.com/en/e-book/354544/how-can-we-move-away-from-vertical-to-horizontal-health-programs

Jenkins Tanga

How Can We Move Away from Vertical to Horizontal Health Programs?

GRIN Publishing

GRIN - Your knowledge has value

Since its foundation in 1998, GRIN has specialized in publishing academic texts by students, college teachers and other academics as e-book and printed book. The website www.grin.com is an ideal platform for presenting term papers, final papers, scientific essays, dissertations and specialist books.

Visit us on the internet:

http://www.grin.com/

http://www.facebook.com/grincom

http://www.twitter.com/grin_com

MSc in Development Studies

How Can We Move Away From Vertical to
Horizontal Health Programs? A Case Study of HIV/AIDS in Uganda

Abstract

This paper examines how governments and health organizations can successfully transit from vertical programming into a broad-based and inclusive community based Primary Health Care that responds to the needs of the local community. Using HIV/AIDS in Uganda as a case study, this paper finds that though these programs are important in combatting some of the biggest pandemics affecting the largest percentage of most populations in the developing world, enhancing the efficacy of vertical programs requires its integration into the more inclusive Primary Health Care system.

TABLE OF CONTENTS

LIST OF ACRONYMNS

3TC	Lamivudine
ABC	Abstinence, Being faithful and Condom use
AEGIS	AIDS Education Global Information System
AIDS	Acquired Immunodeficiency Syndrome
ANC	Antenatal Care
ART	Antiretroviral Therapy
ARV	Antiretroviral Drugs
AZT	Zidovudine
CDC	The US Centers for Disease Control
EFV	Efavirenz
eMTCT	emergency Mother To Child Transmission
HAART	Highly Active Antiretroviral Therapy
HBHTC	Home-based HIV Counselling and Testing
HCT	HIV Counselling and Testing
HIV	Human Immunodeficiency Virus
MCH	Maternal and Child Health
MOH	Ministry of Health (Uganda)
MTCT	Mother To Child Transmission
NCDs	Non-Communicable Diseases
NGO	Non-Governmental Organisation
NVP	Nevirapine
PHC	Primary Health Care
PLWHIV	People Living With HIV/AIDS
RCT	Routine Counselling and Testing
SRH	Sexual Reproductive Health
TDF	Tenofovir
THETA	Traditional & Modern Health Practitioners Together Against AIDS
UNAIDS	Joint United Nations programme on HIV and AIDS
VCT	Voluntary Counselling and Testing
WHO	World Health Organization

CHAPTER ONE:

Introduction and Background.

The course of human history has been deeply affected by infectious diseases. The extent of impact of HIV/AIDS on sub-Saharan African countries has been devastating failing social patterns, healthcare systems and government foundations. HIV/AIDS has over the past 25 years become a part of the modern world with every country reporting and acknowledging the infection amongst its population (Merson, O'Malley, Serwadda, & Apisuk, 2008). This has therefore led to an unprecedented global response that has been termed 'AIDS exceptionalism' where the disease has been seen as requiring a response that is way beyond any normal health intervention (Smith & Whiteside, 2010), thereby attracting a number of stand-alone programs aimed at curbing it. Though some studies link the pandemic to the five cases of pneumonia in gay men in Los Angeles reported by the US Centers for Disease Control and Prevention (Anon, 1981), Faria et al (2014) traces the epidemic way back to the colonial times of the 1920s when the pandemic crisscrossed from the chimpanzees to the humans through hunting and was later fast spread by an active transport network that linked Kinshasa to the rest of sub-Saharan Africa. The CDC initially thought that this disease was confined to homosexual men but this premise was nullified towards the end of 1981 when cases of the disease was reported among non-homosexual injecting drug users in the UK (Merson, O'Malley, Serwadda, & Apisuk, 2008).

The ability of different policy makers in different divisions to network are reduced by vertical programs. This is because health workers and managers are made to remain specialized and isolated because of the competition for limited resources (Lush , 2002). Delivery of HIV/AIDS services is usually done through vertical health programmes. Fragile public health services in resource poor countries are undermined by vertical health programs simply because they divert Health Care Workers (HCW) and other resources away from other programs (Dambisya et al., 2009). The enthusiasim of addressing the AIDS pandemic has created various negtive effects due to vertical programming such as wage distortions, dramatic escalation, unsustainable demands on the health workforce, thereby dwarfing national health budgets because of external funding (Levine, 2007). In a study done in Mozambique, it was noted that excessive funding caused by external funding starved the ministry of support of administrative functions as there was a massive movement of workers from the public sector to private international and private organisations, because funding was channeled through the non-profit organisations (Mussa et al., 2013).

The concept of Primary Health Care has had a massive impact on health practitioners in various developing countries with many not understanding the origins of the term. As cold war was coming to an end (late 1960s and early 1970s), the political context of the US being entangled in a crisis of its own world hegemony, gave rise to the concept of Primary Health Care, keeping in mind that this was a time when the vertical approach used by the US and WHO in combatting malaria in the late 1950s, was under heavy criticism (Cueto, 2004). In 1975, a joint WHO-UNICEF report titled 'Alternative Approaches to Meeting Basic Health Needs in Developing Countries' was released with the term 'Alternative' meaning the shortcomings of traditional vertical programs' concentration on specific diseases (ibid). In 1978, the Alma-Ata Declaration noted the importance of a comprehensive community-oriented comprehensive PHC for all states. WHO launched an initiative of 'Health for All by 2000' after Alma-Ata and it based on the principle of a horizontal mode of delivery of basic health services (WHO, Primary Health Care: Report of the International Conference on Primary Health Care, Alma-Ata 1978, 1978). Termed as comprehensive or horizontal generally means that healthcare is seen as a basic human right that involves the community as community participation is needed for it to become a reality.

Some critiques like Walsh and Warren were skeptical of the concept of comprehensive healthcare arguing that this was a concept not meant for developing countries, as it was unattainable because of the high costs needed to run it such as large numbers of trained personnel and prohibitive costs, thereby initiating a new appealing concept of 'selective PHC', an approach aimed at concentrating on the greatest disease burden of the country (Walsh & Warren, 1980). Vertical programs therefore aim at solving a specific health problem with the application of selective measures but it should be noted that this type of approach is based on the short-term look. Vertical health programs move around the premise that in resource limited settings, health planners are better off prioritizing their interventions (Msuya, 2003). This differs from the comprehensive approach that aims at constructing permanent institutional infrastructure to handle general health services thus tackling overall health problems with a long term process (Maeseneer, et al., 2008).

To move away from the vertical health programs, we need to integrate these programs hence making them comprehensive (horizontal) thereby improving Primary Health Care in general. Integration as a concept in health has various meanings such as training of personnel to provide multiple services, provision of tools, processes and training to better link separate services, harmonization of logistics systems such as data collection, transport and supervision across services, drug and maternal distribution (Pfeiffer, et al., 2010). World Health Organization defines it as "The management and delivery of health services so that clients receive a continuum of preventive and curative services, according to their needs over time and across different levels of the health system." (WHO, 2008). However, for the purpose of this research paper, I will look at integration as the provision of HIV services and programs with other health services at a single point of access or by using referrals within a single health region.

The study uses HIV/AIDS in Uganda as a case study because Uganda has often stood out in the world as one of the earliest, convincing and success models in the fight against HIV/AIDS. Since the early 1980s, HIV has had a stern impact on Uganda. Starting in Rakai district located in the South Western part of the country, HIV eventually spread to the whole country. A strange 'wasting disease' started to claim the lives of people in Rakai district and by 1982 became known as 'slim' though no one had associated the evidence with what would later be known as HIV. It was not until the late 1983 and early 1984 that a team of Ugandan and foreign doctors including Dr. David Serwadda working at the Uganda Cancer Institute in Mulago Hospital National Referral Hospital and Dr. J. Wilson Carsell, a British surgeon observed repeated evidence of Karposi's Sarcoma among young patients all from Rakai district who sent blood samples to Robert Downing at the Centre for Applied Microbiological Research, at Portion Down in the UK who confirmed it was HIV-1 as originally labelled (Putzel, 2004). Major urban areas and along highways necessitated the quick spread of HIV infection to all districts in the country by 1986, acquiring the term generalized epidemic that left many families annihilated, necessitating the rise to a wave of AIDS as an increased number of people were succumbing to infections rising out of their weak immune system (MOH & ORC Macro, Uganda HIV/AIDS Sero-behavioural Survey 2004-2005, 2006). Because of the economic collapse and social dislocation existent at the time, new economic activities materialized. Young women turned to sex trade situating themselves on highways.

This was because at the time, disposable income was with long distance truckers who were often away from home and this gave rise to brothels and bars along the routes in search of income generating activities, and so the unregulated commercial sex work and multiple sexual partners along the routes facilitated the rise and spread of AIDS (Putzel, 2004). Putzel (2004), goes on to note that warfare and social movement also played a role in the spread of HIV and so the combined effects of the social, political and economic disruption and war necessitated the spread of the virus from high risk groups like soldiers, truckers and commercial sex workers to the general population. After the capturing of power by Y.K Museveni's NRM, a national open minded and aggressive stand that involved international, local, national and individuals coming together to fight AIDS was deployed which saw a massive decline in prevalence rates i.e. a reported drop in HIV-1 infection rates from 30% in the early 1990s to 10% in 1996 and 6.5% in 2006 played a major role in Uganda's labelled success story (Kiweewa, 2008). However, it should be noted that HIV prevalence of the general population in Uganda increased from 6.4% in 2004/5 to approximately 7.4% in 2012/13 which strongly undermines the earlier interventions that reduced the prevalence rates in the earlier years (Uganda Aids Commission, 2015). But this can be attributed to the over reliance of ART that has reduced on the number of deaths ie ART increased from 330,000 in 2011 to approximately 750,896 in 2014 hence reducing HIV related deaths from 67000 in 2011 to 31000 in 2014 (ibid).

An unprecedented increase of financial support over the years has been noted to go into developing countries. Only disadvantage is that regardless of the positive development, allocation of these funds tends to focus on disease-specific projects dubbed 'vertical programs' as opposed to more broad based improvements in population health such as primary care services, preventive measures and health workforce development known as 'horizontal programming,' for instance Clinton foundations and Bill and Melinda Gates initiatives that deal with particular communicable diseases (Maeseneer, et al., 2008). Already wrestling with huge inflows of foreign money to fund programs such as AIDS, is Uganda with an estimation of over $100 million each year entering the country to run AIDS projects (Fawzia, 2005). This is because the funding for HIV/AIDS in Uganda remains predominantly donor funded, with the government contributing 12%, private sources only 20% and development partners 68% (Uganda Aids Commission, National AIDS Spending Assesment Uganda 2008/9-2009/10, 2012). This therefore signifies the fact that Uganda will have to adhere to the donors' preferences hence initiation of vertical programs.

In Uganda, the PHC concept was seen as a timely innovation and adopted by Uganda after the Alma-Ata conference as the basis of the development of its health system from the establishment of an extensive network of health units and hospitals with health inspectors running the home hygiene and preventive programmes to that of a more community-oriented health service. However, during the period of sensitization of health workers (1980-1983), a debate between comprehensive PHC and selective PHC ensued with selective PHC coming up as a preferred strategy and so vertical projects came up defeating the idea of horizontal holistic implementation of PHC programmes (Tashobya & Ogwal).

Uganda has a number of programs which are categorized under prevention, care & support and treatment aimed at dealing with the HIV/AIDS pandemic. These programs are run by the Uganda government and assisted by some NGOs. These programs are PMTCT, HCT, ART, ABC, OBULAMU campaign program, Mango Tree Program, THETA. Prevention has been the principal reaction in Uganda till to date with a call for a combined prevention approach that includes biomedical interventions (condoms, treatment, needle exchanges, testing and PMTCT), behavioral interventions (sex education, counselling, programs to reduce stigma & discrimination and cash transfer programs) and structural interventions (interventions to address inequality, decriminalization of sex work, homosexuality, drug use, increasing access to school education for young girls, laws protecting the rights of PLWHIV) (AVERT, 2016).

There has been increasing debate on the importance of vertical programming on the improvement of developing weak health systems. This debate hasn't excluded HIV/AIDS as it attracts a lot of vertical attention thereby leading to debates centering on the premise of whether the over concentration on HIV programs strengthens or weakens fragile health systems. Due to major global health initiatives, increased resources have been brought into countries for HIV programs (Yu, Souteyrand, Banda, Kaufman, & Perriëns, 2008). This has come with advantages such as the heightened consciousness of public health by individual governments, improved and expanded services to PLWHIV and ART provision has enhanced the health of the workforce however, this has led to some very negative impacts such as the stagnation and detoriation of SRH services and general health services (ibid, 2008).

Politics of AIDS

The impact of HIV/AIDS in the world today can be clearly seen as a reflection of the Bubonic plague that hit Europe many years ago. By the closure of 2015, UNAIDS estimations of PLWHIV globally stood at 36.7 million (UNAIDS, Global AIDS Update, 2016) with the majority of infections coming from sub-Saharan Africa standing at 25.5 million. This has led to the rise of responses that have a sort of predominant pattern. This thereby has led to a number of responses that have been inadequate in Africa and this can be attributed to the weak fragile states and the infliction of prevention strategies that are unfamiliar with the cultures and traditions of Africa.

The eradication of AIDS has been separated into three main lines notably politics, economics and weak fragile states. The political dimension which has been propagated by Van der Vliet sees the best way of dealing with the disease as promoting sex education and behavioral change but this may affect some political groupings which would de-campaign this initiative in favor of their own goals (Van der Vliet, 1994). The economics argument is raised by Poku & Whiteside who blame the insufficiency of HIV response in Africa on the various socio-economic crises affecting African countries such as poverty, famine and weak fiscal policies (Poku & Whiteside, 2004). Nevertheless, Patterson looks at the nature of the African state being weak as the reason behind the inadequacy of the programs noting that the state lacks leadership, resources and associations that will enable it fend off the disease (Patterson, 2005).

The most striking argument is the political dimension because it resonates the rights based approach and the principle of paternalism which portrays vulnerability mixed with control (Barnett, 2012). This kind of outlook is a manifestation of the creation of Western knowledge that portrays other huge regions of the world as being disease-prone & poor, inferior & incapable thereby giving Western medicines and pre-emptive structures the capability to deal with these epidemics (Bankoff, 2001). This has therefore led to the transfer of Western models that ignore the African cultures and traditions. This thereby portrays the over-reliance on implementation of drugs and policies as the reason for the inadequacy of HIV response in Africa as a cover-up to the bigger picture of the realm of power politics. This thereby acknowledges the fact that responses to the pandemic shouldn't be separated from the socio-political economic history and structure of the African state.

However, regardless of the fact that the problems concerning the eradication of HIV/AIDS are way beyond vertical programming and policies, this research carries importance into adding to our understanding of the importance of integrating vertical health systems into Primary and comprehensive Health Care system using the case study of HIV/AIDS in Uganda.

This dissertation gathers incentive from the need to scrutinize how governments of developing countries can shift away from vertical programming and programs answering the questions: Has Uganda started to integrate the vertical programs? If it has integrated some of these programs, why has it done so and how can it improve the integration based on evidence? If it hasn't integrated some of these programs, what can be done to integrate these programs based on evidence? To answer these questions, this dissertation will use three standard HIV programs notably PMTCT, HCT and ART.

In order to articulately answer these research questions, this dissertation is further structured as follows. Chapter Two lays emphasis on the methodology used in this dissertation, Chapter Three undertakes an analysis of the three chosen programs of PMTCT, HCT, and ART which will then take this research to its final Chapter Four that will contain the conclusion.

CHAPTER TWO:

Methodology

This research will adopt a case study investigative approach to scrutinize and elucidate how the concept of vertical programs can be transformed into a more beneficial comprehensive health care system approach. In order to gain a thorough appreciation of an issue, event or phenomenon of interest in its natural real-life context, a case study approach is of salient importance (Crowe, et al., 2011).

For the purposes of this study, a wide-ranging examination of peer reviewed academic articles, policy documents, reports and grey literature were used. The search approach used necessitated the usage of a mixed approach which involved the use of search terms such as "HIV/AIDS in Uganda", "HIV programs in Uganda", "Vertical programs", Primary Health Care or Comprehensive Health Systems", "Integration", and the non-use of search terms because at times these search terms could have been used inversely. This therefore required the scrutiny of service provision so as to find out if it fulfilled the criteria of this paper's definition of integration.

Various databases were searched such as PubMed, The Lancet, Google Scholar, Ministry of Health Uganda library, World Health Organization library, UNAIDS library, POPLINE, BioMed central, AEGIS as well as books, non-academic articles and internet sources. The bibliography of the relevant included studies were also vetted in order to get more articles that were relevant to the study.

This chapter contains an analysis of the three chosen programs in order to ascertain if they are integrated or not, why they were integrated if they are integrated and recommendations on how they can be made better if they are integrated or on how they can integrate them into the comprehensive health system if they are not integrated.

PMTCT

Background

The UN General Assembly in 2001 set an 80% target for pregnant women and their children to have access to vital prevention, treatment and care by 2010 to lessen the percentage of infants affected by HIV by 50% (World Health Organisation, 2010). MTCT which is the second largest mode of HIV transmission worldwide, occurs mostly in the developing world more so sub-Saharan Africa where PMTCT though promising, still is a complex and challenging programmatic undertaking (Hladik, Stover, Esiru, Herper, & Trappero, 2009). In 2002, when UNICEF carried out experimental studies in 11 countries including Uganda, it became clear that the implementation of PMTCT was not to be as easy, as it was found that over half of the women who were HIV positive had not ever received antiretroviral treatment (UNICEF, 2003). In 2010, a UN review of its progress found that in sub-Saharan Africa, only 53% of women living with HIV had received anti-retroviral drugs to prevent MTCT (WHO,UNAIDS,UNICEF, 2010).

This therefore initiated a renewed UN commitment to ensure that information, counselling, access to antenatal care and other HIV services were made available to pregnant women (UN, 2011). A three pillar strategy was initially put forward by WHO and UNAIDS notably to prevent i) new infections among parents, ii) unwanted pregnancies among HIV infected women and iii) transmission from HIV-infected pregnant women and mothers to children but later a fourth was added i.e. to provide care and support to mothers, their infants and their families (WHO, Strategic approaches to the prevention of HIV infection in infants: report of a WHO Meeting., 2002).

This therefore made PMTCT a four pronged strategy. As noted by the MOH, MTCT is viewed as the second main mode of HIV transmission in Uganda and the main source of transmission to children (MOH, The Integrated National Guidelines on Antiretroviral Therapy, Prevention of Mother To Child Transmission of HIV, Infant and Young Child Feeding, 2012). The year 2000 marked the beginning of a model PMTCT program in Uganda which initially started in 5 referral hospitals in 3 districts (Mbazzi, et al., 2013). Initially initiated under the VCT approach where the initiative to test was upon the client, it later changed to RCT where this initiative to test switched poles to the providers though leaving clients with the option to either take the test or not to take it (Rujumba, Neema, Tumwine, Tylleskär, & Heggenhougen, 2013). These PMTCT services later expanded at a national basis to all hospitals, all HC IV, 90% of HC III and 11% of HC II (MOH, 2011). The Ugandan government has a goal of ensuring provision of PMTCT services and integration of these services into antenatal care at all health centers (USAID, 2011).

Analysis.

PMTCT in Africa in its early years was primarily seen as a tool to prevent transmission to children but due to the incorporation of ART, this has changed to encompass treatment of HIV positive women as well (Hardon, et al., 2012). This can therefore be attributed to the integration of PMTCT into hospitals, ANC and ART integration into PMTCT hence showing that integration of HIV services comprehensively improves the health system as compared to the ideology of stand-alone programs that don't merge different health services together.

PMTCT as a program in Uganda has amalgamated a number of programs or components e.g. comprehensive antenatal care, infant feeding, counselling and administration of short course anti-retroviral regimen, VCT for HIV during pregnancy, intrapartum and postnatal care (Bajunirwe & Muzoora , 2005). Initially, PMTCT programs which were stand-alone when introduced in the low and middle income countries (Car, et al., 2012), took blood samples from clients and took them to their laboratories for testing therefore requiring that clients return and collect their results which most of the times led to patient drop out hence explaining the high dropout rates. Today with the integration of PMTCT in Uganda, nearly all health facilities use rapid testing kits which release results few minutes after blood sample is taken. All 112 districts in the country by the close of 2013, had at least one health facility running the full scope of PMTCT services (UAC, 2014).

This has further led to the institutionalization of routine HIV testing and counselling as part of antenatal care as an entry point for pregnant women into the PMTCT program in Uganda (Rujumba, Neema, Tumwine, Tylleskär, & Heggenhougen, 2013). Initially initiated under the VCT approach, the initiative to test was upon the clients but this later changed when RCT was introduced, as the initiative to test switched to the providers. This however, left the clients with the option to either take the test or not. Counselling and testing for HIV during

ANC is recommended for all pregnant women by the Ugandan National Policy Guidelines for PMTCT if they don't actively opt out (MOH, 2006). This is because the principle of consent is emphasized by the Ugandan policy (Hardon, et al., 2012). The shift from VCT to RCT prompted the integration of PMTCT into ANC and postpartum health care services, thus increasing the testing rates of women attending ANC e.g. in 2010, with RCT as the dominant approach, 63% of all pregnant women tested for HIV, a dramatic turnaround from 18% in 2005 when it was still under VCT (Rujumba, Neema, Tumwine, Tylleskär, & Heggenhougen, 2013). With the integration of PMTCT into the ANC there was an upsurge in pregnant women who got tested and received their results to 94%, 70,904 pregnant women who were known to be HIV positive were attending ANC for newer pregnancies and the percentage of positive mothers who received ARVs for eMTCT and started option B+ rose to 84% in 2014 (UAC, 2015). This shows that integration does improve service delivery as opposed to stand-alone programs.

The analysis and outcomes aggravate important considerations in the debate on whether vertical programs are helpful to fragile health systems and this calls upon us to reconsider the theoretical establishments of incorporating these stand-alone programs into the health system so as to ensure efficient service delivery. As illustrated, PMTCT is getting fused into the PHC system. Initially as a stand-alone program in which testing and diagnosis centers were different and far apart, required clients to comeback at a later date for their results. This encouraged a high number of dropout cases because patients would travel long distances and it was quite expensive to get to the PMTCT facilities. However, the government realized the need to reduce dropout cases hence prompting the integration of PMTCT into the health facilities so as to ensure that services were brought closer to the people through the improvement of ANC.

Why integration?
PMTCT is quite complex because for its success to be achieved, there has to be sequential interventions such as antenatal care, antiretroviral drugs for the pregnant women, HIV testing, post-partum care along with continued antiretroviral treatment to women within the WHO framework of option B and B+ regimens i.e. ART through the breastfeeding period and ART for life respectively (Larsson, et al., 2015). This therefore prompted the integration of PMTCT, HIV counselling and testing into child birth, postpartum health care services and ANC. HIV care service integration with other general health services turned out to be one of the proven strategies to achieving ideal use by targeted populations (UAC, 2015).

The integration of PMTCT interventions with other health care services improves not only access for women and children but also quality of care through the team work usage of personnel and financial resources. In addition, reduction of stigma experienced by HIV positive people is neccessitated by the implementation of the PMTCT program as a part of routine health care (Car, et al., 2012). Integration will also ensure that treatment of infants born to HIV positve mothers is brought closer to patients. Upon the commencement of labor and within 72 hours of birth, nevirapine is orally administered to mothers and infants respectively in order to prevent vertical transmission (Guay, et al., 1999), so the timely response and availability of the ARV drugs is improved by the integration of PMTCT into the health facilities.

Treatment of pregnant women living with HIV and their newborns using a single dose of NVP which is given to the mother during labor and infant within 72 hours of birth, is one of the most effective interventions for PMTCT (Barigye, et al., 2010). However, a major setback to PMTCT has always been the failure of pregnant women who have HIV to return for NVP and so NVP needed to be offered at the time of diagnosis (ibid) thus prompting the integration of PMTCT into ANC as opposed to the ideology of it standing alone as a program.

The need for policy makers to fulfill the PMTCT guidelines set by WHO which included staff capacity building, rolling out option B+, conducting eMTCT campaigns and increasing the tracking of pregnant mothers in their communities (Baylor-Uganda, 2014) requires PMTCT to be fused into the health system for easy evaluation hence the call for integration. It should also be noted that in order to attain the full utilization of PMTCT, a well-functioning health system is needed in order to provide noteworthy interventions that build the PMTCT program and a health system full of vertical programs is weakened and fragile because then the handling of health complications won't complement each other as required for sustainable growth hence the need for integration.

With the initiation of the 'Global Plan' in 2011, a goal of 90% reduction of new infant HIV infections and reduction of HIV maternal related deaths by 50% was set by the international community to be achieved by 2015 (UNAIDS, Global Plan Towards the Elimination of New HIV Infections among children by 2015 and Keeping their mothers alive., 2011). As noted by a study that was done in 11 African countries, integration of PMTCT services into the MCH had to be done in order for the goals to be achieved (Keiffer, et al., 2014). Uganda being one of the 21 Global Plan critical focus African countries therefore had to integrate PMTCT into the PHC in order to achieve the set goals and improve service delivery and efficiency.

Recommendations

The MOH should increase and improve HIV testing in antenatal care. A study done in Uganda showed that amongst women seeking ANC, what determined being tested for HIV was if the facility offered onsite HIV testing (Larsson, et al., 2012). Therefore as done in Mozambique where all health workers were trained in counselling and testing (Pfeiffer, et al., 2010), the same should be done in Uganda as PMTCT efficiency and effectiveness is improved by increasing HIV testing coverage.

PMTCT should include other tropical diseases and STD testing such as malaria prevention through distribution of mosquito nets and mandatory syphilis testing. This will help with ensuring the prolonged disease free growth of the infant and better health for the mother by preventing the acquisition of malaria and guaranteeing the quick detection of other infections. Just like done in Mozambique where antenatal staff were trained in an incorporated protocol that equipped them with malaria preventive therapy and routine syphilis testing skills (Pfeiffer, et al., 2010), Uganda ought to do the same because infected mothers and their infants are easily susceptible to various infections and diseases.

PMTCT should initiate programs that aim at encouraging male participation through educating them about ANC such as in media and community outreach. This would improve health outcomes for women and their infants if men whose women are pregnant and seeking PMTCT services are involved. A study done in Northern Uganda showed that male participation in ANC increases its use and efficiency (Byamugisha, Tumwine, Semiyaga, & Tylleskär, 2010).

HCT

Background

In the endless bustle towards behavioral change for HIV prevention, HCT stands out as a very effective and efficient tool hence making it an integral part of HIV/AIDS eradication campaign. This takes place in three phases notably pre-test counselling an individual's risk levels to HIV is assessed, taking blood sample and finally the disclosure of results. HCT can be defined as the "process through which an individual undergoes confidential counselling to enable the individual make an informed choice about learning his or her HIV status and to take the appropriate action." (UNFPA & IPPF, 2004). Evidence of the significance of HCT as an effective tool of behavioral change date way back to the 1990's when a peer review study that aimed at assessing the impact of VCT on precarious behavior showed how significant VCT was in influencing behavioral change amongst recipient conflicting heterosexual couples (Higgins, et al., 1991). HCT in Uganda started with the establishment of the AIDS Information center (AIC) whose sole purpose was to provide voluntary HIV testing and counselling. This was initiated as a result of the various awareness and education campaigns in late 1980's that were a manifestation of Uganda's open participatory approach towards the epidemic.

This open approach put massive pressure on the national blood bank as many people flocked the bank in order to donate blood so as to get to know their status and due to the blood bank's inability to offer counselling services as an add on to the testing because it was deemed expensive, various organisations notably MOH AIDS Control Program, Nakasero blood bank, Uganda Virus Research Institute (UVRI), WHO, TASO, Uganda Red Cross, Makerere University Faculty of Social Sciences, USAID, InterAid, and World Learning Inc. came together in endless discussions on a way forward to influence further behavioral change with the end result being the initiation of AIC in February 1990 so as to provide VCT (Alwano-Edyegu, Marum, Wheeler, & Kalema, 1991). This therefore made Uganda a pioneer in VCT as it was the first African country to initiate this strategy (UBOS & Macro International Inc, 2007). It should be noted that there were a few HIV testing services but the chances of finding one that had counselling as well were very slim as there was almost none.

Initially VCT services were provided at the AIC offices and certain designated sites but all were within the capital Kampala where mode of operation was that clients would receive services over a period of two weeks as test results were released after two weeks (Alwano-Edyegu, Marum, Wheeler, & Kalema, 1991). HCT is promoted by prevention programs so as to influence behavioral change in order for people to protect themselves against HIV by letting them know their sero-status as this will tremendously help with reducing new infections and accessing social and medical services (Nsabagasani & Yoder, 2006).

Analysis

Comprehensive HIV care and treatment is started with the admittance through VCT (WHO, 2001). HCT is seen as the entry point to access suitable integrated packages of services for the population basing on the test results i.e. for those who test negative, the services are geared towards enabling the individuals stay negative such as reduction of multiple partners, SMC, correct and consistent condom use and for those who are positive, the package will include PMTCT, linkage to care and treatment, behavior change, opportunistic infection management and condom use as well as family planning which is an integral part of the package (UAC, National HIV&AIDS Strategic Plan 2011/12-2014/15, 2011).

Originally the traditional HCT model was a client oriented (stand-alone) one where the client had to take the initiative upon themselves to get tested and this was done at free-standing clinics whose lone purpose was VCT (Alwano-Edyegu, Marum, Wheeler, & Kalema, 1991). Promotional campaigns were the main source of client attraction and influence (Menzies, et al., 2009). In Uganda with the adoption of HBHTC in 2005 and provider initiated HCT which incorporated in it routine healthcare, HCT is no longer restricted to the standalone clinics (Kyaddondo, Wanyenze, Kinsman, & Hardon, 2012). Provider initiated HCT is highly being incorporated into ANC settings at a national basis. This is in line with WHO's plea to HIV endemic countries to fuse a provider initiated HCT into the health facilities in order to increase peoples' awareness of their status (WHO, Guidance on provider-initiated HIV testing and counseling in health facilities., 2007). With the rise of rapid testing technology, HCT programs have now grown in number, size and maturity with new HCT strategies being adopted that enabled the launch of a provider-based initiated strategy that is being offered to patients in health facilities and mobile units that are offered at the community and home level (Menzies, et al., 2009). This follows up on a study done on a Ugandan community that based on a VCT model that aimed at counselling people the moment they received their results while in their homes was greatly accepted by the people of the community which led to positive results and a rise in testing rates due to this HCT model (Were W. , Mermin, Bunnell, Ekwaru, & Kaharuza, 2003).

With the integration, came other public health approach initiatives aimed at bringing counselling closer to the community and further integrating it into the PHC notably HBHTC services. Under this umbrella were door to door services and household member HCT. Door to door services entailed community mobilizers working hand in hand with mobile teams where the mobile teams move to households and offer HCT services and community mobilizers come in to ensure that all households in the area code are visited (Menzies, et al., 2009). Household member HCT is quite comparable to the door to door service, only difference is that in this case they only go to the homes of those who are HIV positive or initiating ART and target the family members (Were W. A., et al., 2006). These findings therefore cast doubt on the ability of vertical programs the service delivery and hence we ought to integrate them in order to move away from this ideology of vertical programming.

Further need for integration of HCT services by the government of Uganda has led to the introduction of routine testing and counselling, diagnostic HTC and mandatory HIV testing in clinical setting. Routine testing and counselling is meant to be part and parcel of other services health facilities offer regardless of the illness at hand, diagnostic HCT where testing is offered by providers to patients who haven't given consent in order to help them with making right decisions about their care, mandatory HIV testing that doesn't require the consent of the patient in the case of tissue donation, post-exposure that raises the need for prophylaxis and for medical legal circumstances such as rape and defilement (MOH, Uganda National Policy Guidelines for HIV Counselling and Testing, 2005) thereby showing that the government is shifting from these once vertical HIV programs by assimilating them into the health system.

As illustrated above, the analysis incites some serious thoughts on the need to shift from stand-alone programs. We have seen that the once vertical program of HCT in Uganda that started with the initiation of VCT in 1990 though helpful in the fight against HIV/AIDS was not as effective. Cases such as this prompted WHO to come up with an integration policy so as to encourage the efficiency of HIV Counselling and Testing. In Uganda the need to meet this policy, led to the development of public health approaches that aimed at incorporating HCT into the PHC system. This necessity led to the instigation of a provider initiated model which meant that HCT was now to be part and parcel of health facility services, which were offered at a single point when patients sought medical care regardless of the illness. This model was comprised of both hospital and community strategies notably Routine Counselling and Testing, Door to Door counseling and testing, household member HCT, mandatory HIV testing and diagnostic HCT. The integration of this once vertical program has helped a great deal with the improvement of the population's general health. This therefore goes on to challenge the ideology of vertical programming as model that can improve service delivery and general health of the population hence supporting that in order for service delivery to be improved, vertical programs have to be integrated.

Why Integrate?

The integration of HCT will ensure the wide-ranging care of all patients. WHO stipulates that in order for Provider Initiated HCT to be successful, it ought to be applied under a supportive framework which involves making sure that adequate resources are available and there is easy connection of patients with all round prevention, care and treatment services (WHO, Guidance on provider-initiated HIV testing and counseling in health facilities., 2007). In order to fulfill this, integration of HIV services into the health system has to take place because it's quite costly running stand-alone programs and also the funding gotten for HIV services as is the case with Uganda can be transferred and utilized to uplift other health sectors through resource pooling.

The acceptance and effectiveness of VCT is hindered by the absence of HIV care and treatment including access to condoms, ART, prophylaxis for PMTCT and treatment for opportunistic infections (Denison, O'Reilly, Schmid, Kennedy, & Sweat, 2008).Under Provider Initiated model, HCT is considered as a standardized procedure of the health facilities. This makes possible the ability to identify other complications and infections that would have propped up basing on the knowledge of one's HIV status because HIV weakens the immune system (ibid) hence justifying the need for single access point service delivery.

Integration of HCT will also ensure that all groups of the population are reached hence comprehensively elevating the general health. Often, HCT has predominantly focused on the HIV positive and as a case segregates those who are negative and yet they are equally as important to the cause of reducing the epidemic. With integration, they too will be covered because with the provision of HCT at a single point will guarantee that both the HIV positive and negative are reached. Integration of HCT will also help with the reduction of stigma, a problem that has always hindered the full utilization of this HIV care service.

Recommendations.

Hindering the total integration of HCT is provider burnout. Due to the heightened demands caused by the up scaling of ANC, there is a lot of work load on the experienced current staff. In this case, just as done in Zimbabwe, the use of lay counsellors where ordinary people from the community working for the local organisations were picked out and trained to be counsellors (Shetty, et al., 2005), Uganda too should borrow and implement this initiative as this would further promote the community participation in matters pertaining their own lives and generally improve on their primary health conditions. These counsellors can help with pre-test and post-test counselling of the negative clients hence leaving the positive ones to the experienced staff hence reducing on the work load. This would also help with prioritizing those who test HIV negative as they have often been left out. A study done in Uganda found that posttest counselling and support received by women who had tested negative was marred by inadequacy (Rujumba, Neema, Tumwine, Tylleskär, & Heggenhougen, 2013). The training of lay counsellors would therefore help a great deal in cutting on this work load and improve service delivery efficiency.

HCT should aim at involving more men through more gender specific sensitization programs and more male user friendly services at the ANC wards in hospitals. This is because the full utilization of this service in Uganda is highly dependent on the men simply because men are the heads of households and thus have control over the resources and decision. This therefore shows that in order for Uganda to achieve better results in HIV prevention, getting men to actively participate is of valued importance. A study done in Uganda showed that VCT use amidst men was quite low and so they are not entirely involved in HIV prevention programs (Bwambale, Ssali, Byaruhanga, Kalyango, & Karamagi, 2008) hence signifying the importance of the participation of both partners in order to make HCT more efficient and effective.

The government should also aim at re-training the counsellors in order to bring them to par with the new HIV prevention and treatment technologies and also help them learn how to handle some complicated situations through initiatives such as counsellor support groups. A study done in Uganda showed stress associated with counselling brought about by situations such as disclosing to first time pregnant women their HIV positive results as one of the main barriers faced by the counsellors (Medley & Kennedy, 2010). Counsellor support groups will therefore help reduce on this as it will mean keeping up to date with the new interventions and expert moral support for the counsellors.

ART

Background
ART is comprised of the use of drug treatments known as ARVs to fight the HIV virus. It should further be noted that the use of at least three ARV drugs to extremely subdue the virus and halt its development is considered standard ART. In sub-Saharan Africa since 1996, Uganda has pioneered the usage of ART, where initially, ARVs which were imported, were distributed to patients who could afford to buy them (Hardon, et al., 2006). The clampdown of viral reproduction is considered the principal objective of ART (Maenza & Flexner, 1998). The cost of ARVs was reduced through the combined initiatives of international organisations such as UNAIDS and private organizations such as the Joint Clinical Research

Centre (JCRC), which imported cheaper generic drugs into the country thereby forcing pharmaceutical companies to cut the prices of some patented ARVs (Hardon, et al., 2006).

In collaboration with the joint United Nations Programme on HIV/AIDS, the government of Uganda embarked on an effort to make available access to ART which was launched in 1997 under the project UNAIDS HIV Drug Access Initiative (Okero, Aceng, Madraa, Namagala, & Serutoke, 2003). The induction of relevant changes in the health care system to improve HIV/AIDS care access inclusive of ART was the purpose of the Drug Access Initiative (Ibid). Terms of agreement for the UNAIDS HIV Drug Access Initiative were developed between UNAIDS and the Government of Uganda and this included hiring a project coordinator, with the initiative establishing National Treatment Guidelines, developing information materials and training and educating health care providers on AIDS care (Weidle, et al., 2002). Authorization to provide ART through the initiative was given to five health care facilities all of which were within and around the capital Kampala, which health facilities had to have a laboratory, counselling services, trained medical staff, secure drug storage and adequate resources for acquisition of the first installment of drugs (Ibid).

The Uganda Ministry of Health presumed lone responsibility for handling access to ART from 2000 with an expansion plan to intensify access to ART in mind, which plan was to be supported by WHO i.e. National Strategic Framework for Expansion of HIV/AIDS care and support in Uganda from 2001/02 to 2005/06 (MOH, The National Strategic Framework for Expansion of HIV/AIDS Care & Support in Uganda, 2001/2–2005/6, 2002). The Ministry of Health in 2003 committed itself to a free ARV treatment plan which started in 2004 in 25 accredited centers and this greatly helped with providing access to the rural population (Nakiyemba , Kwasa , & Akurut, n.d). Non-governmental organisations have also come in to back up the government facilities in providing ART such as The AIDS Support Organisation (TASO), JCRC, Avert, Baylor Uganda, Mildmay Uganda among many others. Uganda has three lines ART regimens ie TDF+3TC+EFV for first line regimen, AZT+3TC in case the first line fails and Darunavir/r + Raltegravir (Etravirine) + TDF and 3TC for the third line of regimen (Riolexus, 2014).

Analysis

In line with Uganda's adopted strategy of incorporating treatment into prevention, the need to raise accessibility of ARVs to those diseased or at risk of acquiring HIV eg new born babies, is now higher than ever.

The ARV program is being initiated by the government of Uganda in over 140 accreditated sites notably National Referral hospital (Mulago), all regional referral hospitals, district hospitals and health center IVs which are the rural health units offering primary care (Hardon, et al., 2006). A survey done in Uganda showed that government had deployed a means of getting ART services closer to the community through task shifting where clinical officers and nurses were being given integrated training inorder to handle correctly and monitor the use of ART and this has helped with reaching the population in the resource constrained setting (Leach-Lemens, 2009). This is also in line with the WHO's "3 by 5" initiative in which it aims to deliver ART through a public health approach (Nemes, et al., 2006) and thus makes integration a feasible initiative as a eans of shifting out of vertical programming. There has been a growth of ART from urban clinics to district hospitals and PHC facilities and over time, this will ease HIV care as the accreditated facilities would be near the patients home (ibid).

ART in Uganda has always been a stand alone program dealing with only HIV prevalence and as a fact was pretty expensive as only those who could afford it, could get it but this has gradually changed as it has become more incorporated into the health system with the scientific discovery that treatment can be used as a prevention mechanism and non profit organisations that have brought these ART services closer to the community. ART today has been fused into maternal and health care as its strongly used as a means of prevention of vertical transmission of HIV from mother to child as it is known to reduce CD4 count if initiated early when pregnant women go for ANC in the health centers.

The 2003 Uganda ART policy draft gave leverage to the initiation and expansion of the public sector provision of ART services with increased fairness, in which it doesn't displace existing private initiatives but simply builds on them hence supporting treatment using an effective and efficient logistic system that strengthens the general health care system at large (MOH, 2003). In Uganda, ARVs are not only used for the treatment of infected people but with the scientific discovery of ARVs reducing vertical transmission of HIV, it started to be used for prevention purposes and thus was combined with MCH under PMTCT and also under post-exposure prophylaxis incase of accidental exposure eg rape victims, health personnel hence showing that ART gradually being phased out of its vertical nature and into the general health system through the principle of integration.

The enrollment on ART in Uganda increased by 66% after the roll out of the 2013 WHO ART guidelines and by 2013, Uganda had 1478 health facilities in all 112 districts providing ARV services (Baylor-Uganda, 2014). With integration, Non-government actors like Baylor Uganda came in to offer a helping hand as out of the 1478 health facilities offering ART, Baylor supported 346 with technical assistance (ibid).

To further promote ART incorporation, hospitals such as St. Joseph's Hospital Kitgum opened up an ART clinc (A' clinic) within the hospital premises as a department of the hospital inorder to bring care closer to the local vulnerable population, a wider range of health services to the people at a single point of access and to improve and encourage positive living among the people of Acholi region. This is a project that was initiated in 2005 when there was low VCT and PMTCT rates and high stigma related incidences simply because by the time, many of the HIV services in the region were provided on a stand alone basis separate from the health care facilities. The clinc provides comprehensive HIV prevention, treatment, care and support that is participatory in nature where it mitigates the impact of HIV/AIDS in the community through 'expert HIV clients' a term given to infected persons who come out to educate the community on the value and possibility of positive living, with children as well trained to be peer educators and counsellors to their fellow children in ARV adherence (St. Joseph's hospital Kitgum, 2016). With this initiative, the hospital engages community based organisations as well in areas of supportive ART adherence and general behavioural health change hence uplifting the community health in general hence delivering ART through a public health approach. Subsequently, the amalgamation of ART into health system has changed HIV treatment, prevention and PHC because it has led to vivid cutbacks in the morbidity and mortality rates and improved health care utilization thereby supporting the point that vertical programs shouldn't just be pushed away with but rather integrated into the PHC system.

As demonstrated above, the analysis raises some provoking questions about the feasibility of vertical programs in combatting serious health infections while improving service delivery and the health system. ART was vertical in nature and was initially provided on a solo basis in which clinics that offered this service were different from the health facilities. Looking at how the administration of ART has been evolving, we have gotten to see that the Government of Uganda realized that in order to shift away from its vertical nature and to scale up the use of ART, it had to fuse ART provision into the existing health system so as for it to be closer to the community and available at the health facilities. Today, ART is provided within the confinements of health facilities and administered with the other health services such as pediatric health care and this has not only brought services closer to the community but has also led to better ART coverage among those HIV positive, reduced the rise of new infections and played a massive role in ensuring that more HIV positive mothers live through birth. This integration also ensures that children born to positive mothers can live better lives by being HIV negative because it reduces the vertical transmission of the HIV from mother to child when administered during labor to the mother and immediately after birth to the new born child.

Why integrate?

The HIV/AIDS universal response started out as an emergency response to the crucial need for prevention and treatment efforts due to the crises of high infections and death rates (Yu, Souteyrand, Banda, Kaufman, & Perriëns, 2008). However, because AIDS is a chronic disease, effective prevention, treatment and care for HIV/AIDS ought to be integrated with the existing health service and system (ibid). Furthermore, integration will move along with WHO's proposed public health approach to ART that looks to scale up access to treatment for HIV positive people involving basic standard treatment procedures and decentralized service delivery, a system upon which Uganda's health system already operates. WHO realized that in resource limited countries, the Western model of specialist physician management and advanced laboratory monitoring just wasn't achievable in their goal to reach a large number of HIV positive children and adults and so decided to deliver treatment through the public and private sector (Gilks, et al., 2006). This thereby influenced their call for integration so as to reach a number of infected people.

Integration also helps with the improvement of the MCH. Maternal and Child Health is one of the pillars upon which Uganda's PHC system is centered so with the assimilation of ART into Maternal and Child Health services and ensuring that they are delivered at a single point is of salient significance to the raising of the general health of the population. It should also be noted integration helps with the expansion of HAART which is essential for the full utilization of HIV care and services as this would improve patients' outcome hence the need for integration.

Recommendations.

However, ART scale up in Uganda is still lacking as ART is still vertical in nature. To improve the integration of ART, the government has to further embrace the public health approach and train nurses, mid-wives and even the family members of the patients to encourage ART adherence. The case of Botswana is a perfect example as they aimed at encouraging a home-based and community based ART delivery approach in order to lessen congestion at health facilities by training nurses to carry out the doctor's work while the lay health workers and community workers fill the gap left by the nurses by doing their work (Wendo, 2005). With this approach, patients are not offered different pills to take but rather combination drugs, with the view point that qualification doesn't really matter if a good diagnosis is made and counselling is good enough to ensure that the patients follow the drug prescriptions, in this way filling the gap left by the human resource constrain (Ibid).

Subsequently what Uganda needs to do is to guarantee that they prepare individuals from the public to go about as social workers and help with the peer education in order to urge compliance to ARV and if condition gets out of hand, they allude the patients to health facilities for further treatment. It should be noted that this is already underway in some health facilities e.g. ST. Joseph's Hospital Kitgum as shown above but what is being advocated for here, is a more intensified version of this so as for the approach to get quicker national level exposure.

CHAPTER FOUR:

Conclusion.

All in all, as seen with the Uganda HIV/AIDS case study, in order to move away from vertical health programs, we need to integrate them into the health system. Health systems in developing countries ought to turn into client perspective based systems leaning towards both acute illness and chronic care because of the persisting infectious diseases like HIV/AIDS and the developing NCDs and what better way to do this than to integrate these vertical programs into the health system (Yu, Souteyrand, Banda, Kaufman, & Perriëns, 2008). Uganda's PHC system is currently centered on MCH, Family Planning, HIV/AIDS and care for episodic and acute illnesses such as the immunisable diseases and so equipping the health system with the skills to handle chronic diseases is of notable advantage hence the need for integration.

People living with HIV often suffer from other health complications and so the integration of vertical HIV services with PHC and SRH services gives chance to the rise of a more patient centered approach. With integration, the PHC system is better equipped to test and diagnose more clients, prevent better the vertical transmission of the disease, improve on follow up cases and enroll more patients into treatment not pushing aside the fact that coverage will greatly be expanded as compared to a stand-alone vertical model. As noted in a study done in Uganda where a family centered approach adopted by mildmay integrated pediatric early diagnosis, prevention, treatment and care into out-patient and in-patient care, maternal and child health services and HIV care led to a substantial increase in demand for and usage of pediatric HIV care (Luyirika, et al., 2013) therefore generally shows that integration improves the health system.

As noted by Lindegren , et al., (2012), integration of these HIV services with maternal, neo-natal, child health and nutrition services including family planning improves on the efficiency, cost effectiveness of coverage of the services as opposed to offering these services separately. Furthermore, services being offered by the same facility will help improve the acceptability and uptake of services while strengthening the existing health care systems overall through the improvement of laboratory services, quality of care, clinical training and stigma among PLWHIV (ibid).

The integration of these health programs will also help with the mobilization of the community to actively participate in the improvement of their own health. HIV programs have often had disappointing outcomes because of their lack of effective community mobilization (Campbell & Cornish, 2010). This can be blamed on its initially stand-alone nature that ignored the fact that community mobilization is of importance because it enables the empowerment of AIDS affected communities to take ahold of their own health. Integration hence increases the possibility that members of the community will engage in health enhancing behavioral change.

The government of Uganda acknowledged the fact that integration still was a challenge as the integration of family planning, primary HIV prevention and long term family HIV/AIDS care and ART into other services was still low, this thereby prompted a new HIV prevention strategy which was initiated in 2011 that aimed at integration of HIV services, SRH and other health services (UAC, National HIV Prevention Strategy 2011-2015, 2011). This can be accredited to the reason as to why Uganda was acknowledged as one of the 21 African countries that tremendously met the goals set by the Global Plan towards the elimination of new infections among children by 2015 and keeping their mothers alive. Uganda was recognized as having the highest improvement in the reduction of new infections among children with a reduction rate of 86%, ensuring that 95% of women living with HIV had access to ARV medicines, reduced final MTCT rate to below 5% standing at 2.9% (UNAIDS, On the Fast Track to an AIDS-Free Generation, 2016).

This paper has argued for the integration of vertical health programs into the PHC system as it's the best way to shift away from stand-alone programs and encourage community mobilization and participation. As discussed, HIV services in Uganda have been integrated into MCH and other health services but a lot more has to be done by the government to integrate these HIV services further into Family Planning and SRH in order to influence further behavioral change and reach ultimate elimination of new infections. However, the integration of HIV services doesn't only rotate around support from policy makers and donors but also local managerial resources, motivated and available service providers to adequately train all medical personnel (Larsson, et al., 2015).

Bibliography

Alwano-Edyegu, M. G., Marum, E., Wheeler, M., & Kalema, S. (1991). *Knowledge is power: Voluntary HIV counselling and testing in Uganda.* Geneva: UNAIDS.

Anon. (1981). Pneumocystis Pneumonia-Los Angeles. *MMWR Morb Mortal Wkly Rep, 30*, 250-52.

AVERT. (2016, August 1). *HIV Prevention Programmes Overview.* Retrieved from AVERT: AVERTing HIV and AIDS: http://www.avert.org/professionals/hiv-programming/prevention/overview

Bajunirwe, F., & Muzoora , M. (2005). Barriers to the implementation of programs for the prevention of mother to child transmission of HIV: A cross-sectional survey in rural and urban Uganda. *AIDS Research and Therapy, 2*(10). doi:10.1186/1742-6405-2-10

Bankoff, G. (2001). Rendering the World Safe: Vulnerability as Western Discourse. *Disasters, 25*(1), 19-35.

Barigye, H., Levin, J., Maher, D., Tindiwegi, G., Atuhumuza, E., Nakibinge, S., & Grosskurth, H. (2010). Operational evaluation of a service for prevention of mother-to-child transmission of HIV in rural Uganda: barriers to uptake of single-dose nevirapine and the role of birth reporting. *Tropical Medicine and International Health, 15*, 1163–1171. doi:10.1111/j.1365-3156.2010.02609.x

Barnett, M. N. (2012). International Patternalsm and Humanitarian Governance. *Global Constitutionalism, 1*(3), 485-521.

Baylor-Uganda. (2014). *Annual Report 2013-2014.* Baylor College of Medicine Children's Foundation-Uganda.

Bwambale, F. M., Ssali, S. N., Byaruhanga, S., Kalyango, J. N., & Karamagi, C. A. (2008). Voluntary HIV Counselling and Testing among Men in Rural Western Uganda; Implications for HIV Prevention. *BMC Public Health, 8*(263).

Byamugisha, R., Tumwine, J. K., Semiyaga, N., & Tylleskär, T. (2010). Determinants of male involvement in the prevention of mother-to-child transmission of HIV programme in Eastern Uganda: a cross-sectional survey. *Reproductive Health, 7*(12).

Campbell, C., & Cornish, F. (2010). Towards a "Fourth Generation" of approaches to HIV/AIDS management: Creating contexts for effective community mobilization, AIDS Care. *Psychological and Socio-medical Aspects of AIDS/HIV, 22*(52), 1569-1579.

Car, L. T., Van Velthoven, M. H., Brusamento, S., Elmoniry, H., Car, J., Majeed, A., . . . Atun, R. (2012). Integrating Prevention of Mother-to-Child HIV Transmission Programs to Improve Uptake: A Systematic Review. *PLoS One, 7*(4). doi:10.1371/journal.pone.0035268

Crowe, S., Cresswell, K., Robertson, A., Huby, G., Avery , A., & Sheikh, A. (2011). The Case Study Approach. *BioMed Central, 11*(100).

Cueto, M. (2004). The Origins of Primary Health Care and Selective Health Care. *American Journal of Public Health*, 1864.

Dambisya, Y. M., Modipa, S. I., & Nyazema, N. Z. (2009). *A Review on the Impact of HIV and AIDS Programmes on Health Worker Retention.* University of Limpopo, Equinet, Training and Research Support Centre, University of Namibia and WHO,East,Central and Southern Afrcian Health Community. Retrieved from www.equinetafrica.org/sites/default/files/uploads/documents/DIS71DambisyaHCWAIDS.pdf

Denison, J. A., O'Reilly, K. R., Schmid, G. P., Kennedy, C. E., & Sweat, M. D. (2008). HIV Voluntary Counseling and Testing and Behavioral Risk Reduction in Developing Countries: A Meta-analysis, 1990–2005. *AIDS Behav*, 363–373.

Druce, N., & Nolan, A. (2007). Seizing the Big Missed Opportunity: Linking HIV and Maternity Care Services in Sub-Saharan Africa. *Reproductive Health Matters*, 190-201.

Faria , N. R., Rambaut, A., Suchard, M. A., Baele, G., Bedford, T., Ward, M. J., . . . Lemey, P. (2014). The Early Spread and Epidemic Iginition of HIV-1 in Human Populations. *PMC*, 56-61.

Fawzia, S. (2005, May 2). *Uganda and Foreign Aid*. Retrieved from Worldpress.org: www.worldpress.org/print_article.cfm?article_id=2194&dont=yes

Gilks, C. F., Crowley, S., Ekpini, R., Gove, S., Perriens, J., Souteyran, Y., . . . De Cock, K. (2006). The WHO public-health approach to antiretroviral treatment against HIV in resource-limited settings. *Lancet*, 505-10.

Guay, L. A., Musoke, P., Fleming, T., Bagenda, D., Allen, M., Nakabiito, C., . . . Jackson, B. J. (1999). Intrapartum and neonatal single-dose nevirapine compared with zidovudine for prevention of mother-to-child transmission of HIV-1 in Kampala, Uganda: HIVNET 012 randomised trial. *The Lancet*, 795-802.

Hardon, A., Davey, s., Gerrita, T., Hodgkin, C., Irunde, H., Kgatlwane, J., . . . Laing, R. (2006). *From access to adherence: the challenges of antiretroviral treatment, studies from Botswana, Tanzania and Uganda*. Geneva: World Health Organisation.

Hardon, A., Vernooij, E., Bongololo-Mbera, G., Cherutich, P., Desclaux, A., Kyaddondo, D., . . . Obermeyer, C. (2012). Women's views on consent, counseling and confidentiality in PMTCT: a mixed-methods study in four African countries. *BMC Public Health, 12*(26).

Higgins, D., Galavotti, C., O'Reilly, K., Schnell, D., Moore, M., Rugg, D., & Johnson , R. (1991). Evidence for the effects of HIV antibody counseling and testing on risk behaviors. *JAMA*, 2419-29.

Hladik, W., Stover, J., Esiru, G., Herper, M., & Trappero, J. (2009). The Contribution of Family Planning towards the Prevention of Vertical HIV Transmission in Uganda. *PLosone, 4*(11).

Keiffer, M. P., Mattingly, M., Giphart, A., Van de Ven, R., Chouraya, C., Walakira, M., . . . EGPAF Technical Directors Forum. (2014). Lessons Learned From Early Implementation of Option B+: The Elizabeth Glaser Pediatric AIDS Foundation Experience in 11 African Countries. *J Acquir Immune Defic Syndr*, S188-S194.

Kiweewa, J. M. (2008, November). Uganda's HIV/AIDS success story: Reviewing the Evidence. *Journal of Development and Social Transformation, 5*.

Kyaddondo, D., Wanyenze, R. K., Kinsman, J., & Hardon, A. (2012). Home-based HIV Counselling and Testing: Client Experiences and Perceptions in Eastern Uganda. *BMC Public Health, 12*(966).

Larsson, E. C., Ekstrom, A. M., Pariyo, G., Tomson, G., Sarowar, M., Baluka, R., . . . Thorson, A. E. (2015). Prevention of Mother to Child transmission of HIV in rural Uganda: Modelling effectiveness and impact of scaling up PMTCT services. *Global Health Action*.

Larsson, E., Thorson, A., Pariyo, G., Conrad, P., Arinaitwe , M., & Kemigisa, M. (2012). Opt-out HIV Testing During Antenatal Care: Experiences of Pregnant Women in Rural Uganda. *Health Policy Plan*, 69-75.

Leach-Lemens, C. (2009, September 1). *Uganda survey shows major ART training gaps for non-physicians*. Retrieved from nam aidsmap; HIV&AIDS sharing knowledge, changing lives: http://www.aidsmap.com/Uganda-survey-shows-major-ART-training-gaps-for-non-physicians/page/1435832/

Levine, R. (2007, 05 10). *Should Vertical Health Programs Just Lie Down?* Retrieved from Center For Global Development.: www.cgdev.org/blog/should-all-vertical-programs-just-lie-down

Lindegren , M., Kennedy, C., Bain-Brickley , D., Azman, H., Creanga, A., Butler, L., . . . Kennedy, G. (2012). Integration of HIV/AIDS services with maternal, neonatal and child health, nutrition, and family planning services (Review). *The Cochrane Collaboration*.

Lush , L. (2002, June). *Service Integration: An Overview of Policy Developments*. Retrieved from Guttmacher Institute: www.guttmacher.org/about/journals/ipsrh/2002/06/service-integration-overview-policy-developments

Luyirika, E., Towle, M. S., Achen, J., Muhangi, J., Senyimba, C., Lule, F., & Muhe, L. (2013). Scaling Up Pediatric HIV Care with an Integrated Family-Centered Approach: An Observational Case Study from Uganda. *PLOSone, 8*(8).

Maenza, J., & Flexner, C. (1998). Combination Antiretroviral Therapy for HIV Infection. *Am Fam Physician, 57*(11), 2789-2798.

Maeseneer, J. D., Weel, C. V., Egilman, D., Mfenyana, K., Kaufman, A., & Sewankambo, N. (2008). Strengthening Primary Care: addressing the disparity between vertical and horizontal investment. *The British Journal of General Practice.*, 3-4.

Mbazzi, F. B., Zucca, M. L., Ojom, L., Kabasomi, S. V., Esiru, G., & Homsy, J. (2013). High PMTCT Program Uptake and Coverage of Mothers, Their Partners and Babies in Northern Uganda: Achievements and Lessons Learned Over 10 Years of Implementation (2002-2011). *Acquir Immune Defic Syndr, 62*, 138-145.

Medley, A. M., & Kennedy, C. E. (2010). Provider Challenge in Implementing Antenatal Provider-Initiated HIV Testing and Counselling Programs in Uganda. *AIDS Education and Prevention, 22*(2), 87-99.

Menzies, N., Abang, B., Wanyenzee, R., Nuwaha, F., Mugisha, B., Coutinho, A., . . . Blandford, J. M. (2009). The costs and effectiveness of four HIV counseling and testing strategies in Uganda. *Wolters Kluwer Health*.

Merson, M. H., O'Malley, J., Serwadda, D., & Apisuk, C. (2008). The History and Challenge of HIV Prevention. *The Lancet*, 475-88.

MOH. (2002). *The National Strategic Framework for Expansion of HIV/AIDS Care & Support in Uganda, 2001/2–2005/6*. Kampala: Ministry of Health.

MOH. (2003). *DRAFT ANTIRETROVIRAL TREATMENT POLICY FOR UGANDA*. Kampala: Ministry of Health Uganda.

MOH. (2005). *Uganda National Policy Guidelines for HIV Counselling and Testing*. Kampala: Ministry of Health.

MOH. (2006). *Policy guidelines for prevention of mother-to child transmission.* Kampala: Ministry of Health Uganda.

MOH. (2011). *PMTCT Annual Report .* Kampala: Ministry of Health Uganda.

MOH. (2012). *The Integrated National Guidelines on Antiretroviral Therapy, Prevention of Mother To Child Transmission of HIV, Infant and Young Child Feeding.* Kampala: Ministry Of Health Uganda.

MOH, & ORC Macro. (2006). *Uganda HIV/AIDS Sero-behavioural Survey 2004-2005.* Calverton, Maryland: Ministry of Health and ORC Macro.

Msuya, J. (2003). *Horizontal and Vertical Delivery of Health Services: What are the Trade offs?* Washington DC: World Bank.

Mussa , A. H., Pfeiffer , J., Gloyd , S. S., & Sherr, K. (2013). Vertical Funding, non-governmental organisations and health system strengthening: perspectives of public sector health workers in Mozambique. *Hmn Resour Health.*

Nakiyemba , A., Kwasa , R., & Akurut, D. (n.d.). *Uganda-WHO archives.* Retrieved from World Health Organisation: http://archives.who.int/prduc2004/FinalProposalARVAdherenceStudyUganda.pdf.

Nemes, M. I., Beaudoin, J., Conway, S., Kivumbi, G. W., Skjelmerud, A., & Vogel, U. (2006). *EVALUATION OF WHO's CONTRIBUTION TO "3 BY 5" Main Report.* Geneva: World Health Organisation.

Nsabagasani, X., & Yoder, S. P. (2006). *Social Dynamics of VCT and Disclosure in Uganda.* Calverton, Maryland: UPHOLD Project and Macro International Inc.

Okero, A. F., Aceng, E., Madraa, E., Namagala, E., & Serutoke, J. (2003). *Scaling Up Antiretroviral Therapy: Experience In Uganda.* Geneva: World Health Organization.

Patterson, A. S. (2005). *The African state and the AIDS crisis.* Aldershot: Ashgate Publishing.

Pfeiffer, J., Montoya, P., Baptista, A. J., Karagianis, M., Pugas, M., Micek, M., . . . Gloyd, S. (2010). Integration of HIV/AIDS services into African primary health care: lessons learned for health system strengthening in Mozambique - a case study. *Journal of the International AIDS Society.*

Poku, N. K., & Whiteside, A. (2004). *The Political Economy of AIDS in Africa.* Burlington: Ashgate Publishing .

Press Release. (2007). *The Global Fund, The Focus on three Diseases and the challenges of improving African health services.* GFATM.

Putzel, J. (2004). THE POLITICS OF ACTION ON AIDS: A CASE STUDY OF UGANDA. *Public Admin. Dev, 24,* 19–30. doi:10.1002/pad.306

Riolexus, A. A. (2014, March). *THE NATIONAL ANTIRETROVIRAL TREATMENT GUIDELINES FOR UGANDA 2013.* Retrieved from ATIC Newsletter, Infectious Diseases Institute, Makerere University Kampala: http://www.idi-makerere.com/docs/Atic%20Newsletter_march%20%202014.pdf

Rujumba, J., Neema, S., Tumwine, J. K., Tylleskär, T., & Heggenhougen, H. K. (2013). Pregnant women's experiences of routine counselling and testing for HIV in Eastern Uganda: a qualitative study. *BMC Health Services Research, 13*(189).

Shetty, A., Mhazo, M., Moyo, S., Von Lieven, A., Mateta, P., Katzenstein, D., . . . Basseti, M. (2005). The Feasibility of Voluntary Counselling and HIV Testing For Pregnant Women Using Community Volunteers in Zimbabwe. *Int J STD AIDS, 16*(11), 755-9.

Smith , J. H., & Whiteside, A. (2010). The History of AIDS exceptionalism. *Journal of the International AIDS Society, 13*(47).

St. Joseph's hospital Kitgum. (2016, July 25). *Art Clinic (A' Clinic)* . Retrieved from St. Joseph's hospital Kitgum; Love serve with honesty: http://www.sjhkitgum.org/index.php/departpments/art-clinic-a-clinic

Tashobya, C. K., & Ogwal, P. O. (n.d.). *PRIMARY HEALTH CARE AND HEALTH SECTOR REFORMS IN UGANDA*. Retrieved from http://www.bioline.org.br/pdf?hp04006

UAC. (2011). *National HIV Prevention Strategy 2011-2015*. Kampala: Uganda Aids Commission.

UAC. (2011). *National HIV&AIDS Strategic Plan 2011/12-2014/15*. Kampala: Uganda Aids Commission.

UAC. (2014). *HIV and AIDS Uganda Country Progress Report; 2013*. Kampala: Uganda Aids Commission. Retrieved from http://www.aidsuganda.org

UAC. (2015). *National HIV&AIDS Priority Action Plan 2015/2016-2017/2018*. Kampala: Uganda Aids Commission.

UAC. (2015). *THE HIV AND AIDS UGANDA COUNTRY PROGRESS REPORT 2014*. Kampala: Uganda Aids Commission.

UBOS, & Macro International Inc. (2007). *Uganda Demographic and Health Survey 2006*. Calverton, Maryland: Ubos and Macro International Inc.

Uganda Aids Commission. (2012). *National AIDS Spending Assesment Uganda 2008/9-2009/10*. Kampala: Uganda Aids Commission.

Uganda Aids Commission. (2015). *THE HIV AND AIDS UGANDA COUNTRY PROGRESS REPORT 2014*. Kampala: Uganda Aids Commission.

UN. (2011). *Political declaration on HIV/AIDS: intensifying our efforts to eliminate HIV/AIDS. United Nations general assembly, 65th session, agenda item 10. Resolution adopted by the General assembly on 10th June 2011*. New York: United Nations.

UNAIDS. (2011). *Global Plan Towards the Elimination of New HIV Infections among children by 2015 and Keeping their mothers alive*. Geneva: Joint United Nations programme on HIV/AIDS .

UNAIDS. (2016). *Global AIDS Update*. Geneva: Joint United Nations Programme on HIV/AIDS .

UNAIDS. (2016). *On the Fast Track to an AIDS-Free Generation*. Geneva: Joint United Nations Programme on HIV and AIDS.

UNAIDS, WHO. (2004). *Policy statement on HIv testing* . Geneva: United Nations and World Health Organisation.

UNFPA & IPPF. (2004). *Integrating HIV Voluntary Counselling and Testing Services into Reproductive Health Services*. IPPF South Asia Regional Office and UNFPA.

UNICEF. (2003). *Evaluation of United Nations-supported pilot projects for the Prevention of Mother to Child transmission of HIV*. UNICEF Evaluation Database.

USAID. (2011). *Family Planning and HIV Integration Profile: Uganda.*

Van der Vliet, V. (1994). *The Politics of AIDS.* London: Bowerdean Publishing Co Ltd.

Walsh, J. A., & Warren, K. S. (1980). Selective Primary Healthcare: An Interim Strategy for Disease Control in Developing Countries. *New England Journal at Medicine*, 145-163. Retrieved from http://qmplus.qmul.ac.uk/pluginfile.php/153629/mod_book/chapter/3004/Walsh%20and%20Warren%20PHC.pdf

Weidle, P. J., Malamba, S., Mwebaze, R., Sozi, C., Rukundo, G., Downing, R., . . . Lackritz, E. (2002). Assessment of a pilot antiretroviral drug therapy programme in Uganda: patients' response, survival, and drug resistance. *Lancet*, 34-40.

Wendo, C. (2005, April 4). *Uganda leads way in innovative HIV/AIDS treatment.* Retrieved from World Health Organisation: http://www.who.int/bulletin/volumes/83/4/infocus0405/en/index1.html

Were, W. A., Mermin, J. H., Nafuna, W., Awor, A. C., Bechange, S., Moss, S., . . . Bunnell, R. E. (2006). Undiagnosed HIV Infection and Couple HIV Discordance Among Household Members of HIV-Infected People Receiving Antiretroviral Therapy in Uganda. *J Acquir Immune Defic Syndr*, 91-95.

Were, W., Mermin, J., Bunnell, R., Ekwaru, J. P., & Kaharuza, F. (2003). Home-based Model for HIV Voluntary Counselling and Testing. *The Lancet, 361.* Retrieved from www.thelancet.com

WHO. (1978). *Primary Health Care: Report of the International Conference on Primary Health Care, Alma-Ata 1978.* Geneva: World Health Organisation.

WHO. (2001). *The Health Sector Response to HIV/AIDS; Coverage of selected services in 2001, Preliminary Assessment.* Geneva: World Health Organisation.

WHO. (2002). *Strategic approaches to the prevention of HIV infection in infants: report of a WHO Meeting.* Morges: World Health Organisation.

WHO. (2007). *Guidance on provider-initiated HIV testing and counseling in health facilities.* Geneva: World Health Organisation.

WHO. (2008). *Integrated Health Services- What and Why?* Retrieved from World Health Organization: www.who.int/healthsystems/service_delivery_techbrief1.pdf

WHO,UNAIDS,UNICEF. (2010). *Towards universal access: scaling up priority HIV/AIDS interventions in the health sector: progress report 2010.* Geneva: World Health Organisation.

World Health Organisation. (2010). *PMTCT Strategic vision 2010-2015: Preventing Mother To Child Transmission of HIV to reach the UNGASS and Millenium Development Goals.* Geneva: WHO Press.

Yu, D., Souteyrand, Y., Banda, M. A., Kaufman, J., & Perriëns, J. H. (2008). Investment in HIV/AIDS programs: Does it help strengthen health systems in developing countries? *Globalisation and Health, 4*(8). doi:10.1186/1744-8603-4-8

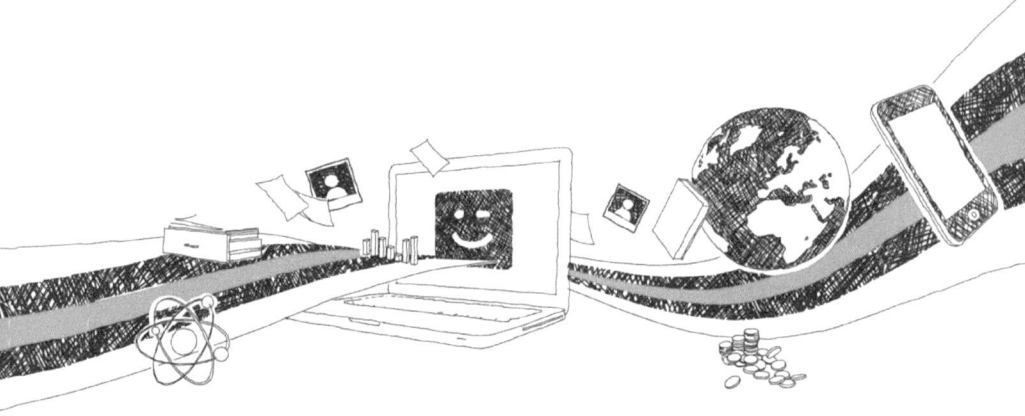
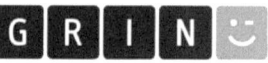